Table of Contents

Chapter 1: Understanding One Meal a Day (OMAD) for Weight Loss

The Basics of OMAD

In this subchapter, we will delve into the basics of OMAD, which stands for One Meal a Day. This eating pattern has gained popularity in recent years as a way to lose weight quickly and effectively. The concept is simple - you eat only one meal a day, typically within a one-hour window, and fast for the remaining 23 hours. This approach can be a powerful tool for weight loss, as it helps to reduce overall calorie intake and regulate hunger hormones.

One of the key benefits of OMAD is its simplicity. Unlike other diets that require complex meal planning and calorie counting, OMAD is straightforward and easy to follow. By eating just one meal a day, you eliminate the need to constantly think about food, which can be a major source of stress for many people trying to lose weight. Additionally, OMAD can help to break unhealthy eating habits and reduce cravings, as you are only allowed to eat during a specific time frame.

It is important to note that OMAD should be done in a healthy way to ensure optimal results. This means focusing on nutrient-dense foods such as fruits, vegetables, lean proteins, and whole grains during your one meal. It is also essential to stay hydrated throughout the day by drinking plenty of water and herbal teas. Additionally, it is recommended to consult with a healthcare professional before starting any new diet or eating plan, especially if you have any underlying health conditions.

Another important aspect of OMAD is listening to your body's hunger cues. It is important to eat until you are comfortably full during your one meal, but not to the point of feeling overly stuffed. This can help to prevent overeating and promote better digestion. It is also important to pay attention to how different foods make you feel and to adjust your meal accordingly to ensure you are getting the nutrients your body needs.

In conclusion, OMAD can be a powerful tool for weight loss when done in a healthy way. By focusing on nutrient-dense foods, staying hydrated, and listening to your body's hunger cues, you can achieve fast and sustainable weight loss results. Remember to consult with a healthcare professional before starting any new eating plan, and to listen to your body throughout the process. With dedication and consistency, OMAD can help you reach your weight loss goals and improve your overall health.

The Science Behind OMAD

In this subchapter, we will delve into the science behind the One Meal a Day (OMAD) approach to weight loss. OMAD is a popular fasting method where individuals consume all their daily calories in just one meal, typically within a one-hour window. This fasting schedule has gained traction in recent years for its potential to promote rapid weight loss and improve overall health.

One of the key scientific principles behind OMAD is the concept of intermittent fasting. By limiting the time window in which you eat to just one meal a day, you are essentially giving your body an extended period of time to rest and repair. During the fasting period, your body switches from using glucose as its primary fuel source to burning stored fat for energy, leading to weight loss.

Research has shown that intermittent fasting, including the OMAD approach, can have numerous benefits beyond weight loss. Studies have found that intermittent fasting can improve insulin sensitivity, reduce inflammation, and promote cellular repair processes. This can lead to a decreased risk of chronic diseases such as type 2 diabetes, heart disease, and cancer.

Furthermore, OMAD can also help regulate hunger hormones such as ghrelin and leptin. When you consume all your calories in one meal, your hunger hormones become more balanced, making it easier to control cravings and reduce overall caloric intake. This can lead to a more sustainable approach to weight loss compared to traditional calorie-restricted diets.

It is important to note that while OMAD can be an effective weight loss strategy, it may not be suitable for everyone. Individuals with certain medical conditions, such as diabetes or eating disorders, should consult with a healthcare professional before embarking on an OMAD regimen. Additionally, it is crucial to ensure that the one meal consumed each day is nutrient-dense and balanced to meet your body's needs for essential vitamins, minerals, and macronutrients.

In conclusion, the science behind OMAD supports its efficacy as a fast weight loss method that can also improve overall health. By understanding the physiological mechanisms at play during intermittent fasting, individuals can make informed decisions about incorporating OMAD into their weight loss journey. As with any dietary approach, it is important to listen to your body's cues and consult with a healthcare provider to ensure that OMAD is a safe and sustainable option for you.

Pros and Cons of OMAD

In the world of weight loss strategies, one that has gained popularity in recent years is OMAD, or One Meal a Day. This approach involves consuming all of your daily calories in just one meal, typically within a one-hour eating window. While some people swear by the effectiveness of OMAD for fast weight loss, others have concerns about its potential drawbacks. In this subchapter, we will explore the pros and cons of OMAD to help you decide if this approach is right for you.

One of the biggest advantages of OMAD is its simplicity. With only one meal to plan and prepare each day, OMAD can save you time and effort in the kitchen. This can be especially appealing for people with busy schedules or limited cooking skills. Additionally, some people find that eating just one meal a day helps them feel more in control of their eating habits and reduces the temptation to snack or overeat.

On the other hand, one of the main concerns with OMAD is the potential for nutrient deficiencies. When you are only eating one meal a day, it can be challenging to get all of the essential nutrients your body needs to function properly. This can lead to deficiencies in vitamins, minerals, and other key nutrients, which can have negative effects on your health in the long term. It is important to carefully plan your OMAD meals to ensure you are getting a balanced and varied diet.

Another potential downside of OMAD is the risk of overeating during your one meal. When you are only eating once a day, there can be a tendency to consume larger portions or high-calorie foods, which can sabotage your weight loss goals. It is important to be mindful of portion sizes and choose nutrient-dense, whole foods to ensure you are meeting your nutritional needs without going overboard on calories.

Despite these drawbacks, many people have found success with OMAD for fast weight loss. By eating just one meal a day, you can create a calorie deficit that can lead to rapid weight loss. Additionally, some studies suggest that intermittent fasting, which includes approaches like OMAD, may have other health benefits such as improved insulin sensitivity and reduced inflammation. If you are considering trying OMAD, it is important to consult with a healthcare provider or nutritionist to ensure you are meeting your nutritional needs and to monitor your progress for any potential negative effects.

Chapter 2: Planning Your One Meal

Creating a Balanced Meal Plan

Creating a balanced meal plan is essential for anyone looking to lose weight fast with the one meal a day approach. It is important to ensure that you are providing your body with all the necessary nutrients it needs to function properly while also creating a calorie deficit to promote weight loss. By following a balanced meal plan, you can fuel your body with the right foods and avoid feeling deprived or fatigued.

When creating a balanced meal plan for weight loss, it is important to focus on including a variety of foods from all the major food groups. This includes incorporating lean proteins, whole grains, fruits, vegetables, and healthy fats into your meals. By including a wide range of foods, you can ensure that you are getting all the essential nutrients your body needs to thrive.

One key aspect of creating a balanced meal plan is to pay attention to portion sizes. It can be easy to overeat when following a one meal a day approach, so it is important to be mindful of the amount of food you are consuming. By portioning out your meals and snacks, you can better control your calorie intake and avoid overeating.

Another important factor to consider when creating a balanced meal plan is to stay hydrated. Drinking plenty of water throughout the day can help keep you feeling full and satisfied, reducing the likelihood of overeating during your one meal. Additionally, staying hydrated can help support your metabolism and promote weight loss.

In conclusion, creating a balanced meal plan is essential for anyone looking to lose weight fast with the one meal a day approach. By focusing on incorporating a variety of foods from all the major food groups, paying attention to portion sizes, and staying hydrated, you can fuel your body with the nutrients it needs while promoting weight loss. Remember to listen to your body's hunger cues and make adjustments to your meal plan as needed to ensure success in your weight loss journey.

Meal Timing and Frequency

Meal timing and frequency play a crucial role in achieving fast weight loss in a healthy way. For people that want to lose weight fast, adopting the practice of consuming one meal a day can be a game-changer. By focusing on eating one nutrient-dense meal a day, you can create a caloric deficit that promotes weight loss while still providing your body with the essential nutrients it needs to function optimally.

One key aspect of meal timing when following a one meal a day approach is to ensure that you are consuming your meal at the same time each day. This consistency helps regulate your body's hunger and satiety signals, making it easier to stick to your eating plan and avoid unnecessary snacking or overeating. By establishing a set mealtime, you can also train your body to expect food at a specific time, reducing cravings and helping you stay on track with your weight loss goals.

In addition to meal timing, the frequency of your meals also plays a significant role in fast weight loss. When following a one meal a day approach, it is essential to focus on the quality of the meal you are consuming. Opt for whole, nutrient-dense foods that provide you with a balance of macronutrients and micronutrients to support your overall health and well-being. Avoid processed and high-sugar foods, as these can sabotage your weight loss efforts and leave you feeling sluggish and hungry.

By eating one meal a day, you give your body time to fully digest and absorb the nutrients from your meal, allowing for optimal energy levels and metabolic function. This can help increase your metabolism and promote fat loss, making it easier to achieve your weight loss goals. Additionally, by focusing on one meal a day, you can develop a healthier relationship with food and learn to listen to your body's hunger cues, leading to long-term sustainable weight loss success.

Overall, meal timing and frequency are essential components of a successful one meal a day weight loss plan. By prioritizing nutrient-dense foods, establishing a consistent mealtime, and focusing on quality over quantity, you can achieve fast weight loss in a healthy and sustainable way. Remember to listen to your body, stay hydrated, and consult with a healthcare professional before making any significant changes to your diet.

Incorporating Nutrient-Dense Foods

One of the key components of successful weight loss is incorporating nutrient-dense foods into your diet. These foods are packed with essential vitamins, minerals, antioxidants, and other beneficial nutrients that are essential for overall health and well-being. By focusing on nutrient-dense foods, you can ensure that you are providing your body with the fuel it needs to function optimally while also supporting your weight loss goals.

When following a one meal a day (OMAD) approach to weight loss, it is especially important to choose nutrient-dense foods that will keep you feeling satisfied and energized throughout the day. Incorporating a variety of fruits, vegetables, whole grains, lean proteins, and healthy fats into your meal can help you meet your nutritional needs while also supporting your weight loss efforts. These foods are not only low in calories but also high in essential nutrients that can help boost your metabolism and support your body's natural detoxification processes.

To ensure that you are getting the most out of your one meal a day, it is important to focus on whole, minimally processed foods. This means avoiding highly processed foods that are high in added sugars, unhealthy fats, and artificial ingredients. Instead, opt for foods that are as close to their natural state as possible, such as fresh fruits and vegetables, whole grains, lean proteins, and healthy fats like avocado, nuts, and seeds.

Incorporating nutrient-dense foods into your one meal a day can help you feel more satisfied and energized, making it easier to stick to your weight loss plan. These foods are also essential for supporting your overall health and well-being, providing your body with the essential nutrients it needs to function optimally. By focusing on nutrient-dense foods, you can ensure that you are getting the most out of your one meal a day while also supporting your weight loss goals in a healthy and sustainable way.

In conclusion, incorporating nutrient-dense foods into your one meal a day can have a significant impact on your weight loss journey. By choosing whole, minimally processed foods that are high in essential nutrients, you can support your body's natural detoxification processes, boost your metabolism, and feel more satisfied and energized throughout the day. Remember to focus on variety and balance in your meal choices to ensure that you are meeting your nutritional needs while also supporting your weight loss goals.

Chapter 3: Implementing OMAD Safely

Consulting with a Healthcare Professional

Consulting with a healthcare professional is a crucial step in embarking on a weight loss journey, especially if you are considering adopting a one meal a day (OMAD) approach to shed those extra pounds. Before making any drastic changes to your diet or lifestyle, it is important to consult with a qualified healthcare professional to ensure that you are making healthy choices that will not harm your body in the long run.

A healthcare professional, such as a doctor or nutritionist, can provide you with personalized guidance and advice based on your individual health needs and goals. They can help you determine if OMAD is a suitable approach for you, taking into consideration factors such as your current weight, medical history, and any underlying health conditions you may have. Consulting with a healthcare professional can also help you identify potential risks and side effects associated with fasting, and develop a plan to mitigate them.

Furthermore, a healthcare professional can help you create a balanced and nutritious meal plan that aligns with your weight loss goals while ensuring that you are still meeting your body's nutritional needs. They can recommend specific foods and portion sizes that will help you stay satisfied and energized throughout the day, even with just one meal. By consulting with a healthcare professional, you can be confident that you are nourishing your body in a way that promotes weight loss without compromising your overall health.

In addition to providing guidance on nutrition and meal planning, a healthcare professional can also offer support and motivation as you work towards your weight loss goals. They can help you set realistic expectations and track your progress over time, offering encouragement and advice to keep you on the right track. Having a healthcare professional by your side can make the weight loss journey feel less daunting and overwhelming, as you will have a trusted expert to turn to for guidance and reassurance.

Overall, consulting with a healthcare professional before starting a one meal a day weight loss plan is essential for ensuring that you are making informed and healthy choices. By working with a qualified professional, you can create a personalized approach to weight loss that is safe, effective, and sustainable in the long term. Remember, your health is the most important thing, so take the time to consult with a healthcare professional before making any changes to your diet or lifestyle.

Listening to Your Body's Signals

When it comes to losing weight fast in a healthy way, one of the most important things you can do is listen to your body's signals. Your body is constantly sending you messages about what it needs, whether it's hungry, thirsty, tired, or in need of movement. By tuning into these signals and responding to them appropriately, you can better support your weight loss goals.

One key signal to pay attention to is hunger. Many people ignore their body's hunger cues and end up overeating or making unhealthy food choices. Instead of waiting until you're starving to eat, try to eat when you start to feel moderately hungry. This can help prevent overeating and keep your energy levels stable throughout the day. Additionally, pay attention to how different foods make you feel. If you notice that certain foods leave you feeling sluggish or bloated, try to avoid them and opt for more nourishing options instead.

Thirst is another important signal that your body sends you. Dehydration can often be mistaken for hunger, leading to unnecessary snacking or overeating. To ensure you're staying hydrated, aim to drink at least eight glasses of water a day. You can also incorporate hydrating foods like fruits and vegetables into your meals to help meet your water needs. By listening to your body's thirst signals and staying properly hydrated, you can support your weight loss efforts and overall health.

In addition to hunger and thirst, your body also sends signals about when it needs rest and movement. Getting an adequate amount of sleep is crucial for weight loss, as lack of sleep has been linked to increased cravings and weight gain. Aim to get at least seven to eight hours of sleep each night to support your weight loss goals. On the flip side, regular movement is also important for weight loss. Find ways to incorporate physical activity into your daily routine, whether it's through walking, biking, or yoga. By listening to your body's signals for rest and movement, you can create a balanced approach to weight loss that supports your overall well-being.

In conclusion, listening to your body's signals is essential for fast and healthy weight loss. By tuning into cues like hunger, thirst, rest, and movement, you can better support your body's needs and make informed choices that align with your weight loss goals. Pay attention to how different foods and activities make you feel, and adjust your habits accordingly. By fostering a deeper connection with your body and its signals, you can achieve sustainable weight loss results that prioritize your health and well-being.

Avoiding Common Mistakes

In the quest to lose weight quickly, it's important to be mindful of common mistakes that can hinder your progress. By avoiding these pitfalls, you can ensure that you are on the right track towards achieving your weight loss goals. Here are some key tips to help you avoid common mistakes when following a one meal a day diet plan.

One common mistake that people make when trying to lose weight fast is skipping meals. While it may seem like a good idea to cut back on calories, skipping meals can actually slow down your metabolism and make it harder for you to lose weight. It's important to eat regular, balanced meals to keep your metabolism running smoothly and to ensure that you are getting the nutrients your body needs to function properly.

Another mistake to avoid when following a one meal a day diet plan is not drinking enough water. Staying hydrated is essential for weight loss, as it helps to boost your metabolism and keep you feeling full. Aim to drink at least eight glasses of water a day, and try to avoid sugary drinks and excessive caffeine, as these can dehydrate you and hinder your weight loss efforts.

It's also important to avoid unhealthy food choices when following a one meal a day diet plan. While it may be tempting to indulge in fast food or processed snacks, these foods are often high in calories and low in nutrients. Instead, focus on eating whole, nutrient-dense foods like fruits, vegetables, lean proteins, and whole grains. These foods will help you feel full and satisfied while providing your body with the essential nutrients it needs to function properly.

Another common mistake to avoid when trying to lose weight fast is not getting enough sleep. Sleep is essential for weight loss, as it helps to regulate your hormones and metabolism. Aim to get at least seven to eight hours of sleep a night, and try to establish a regular sleep schedule to ensure that you are getting enough rest. By prioritizing sleep, you can help to support your weight loss efforts and improve your overall health.

By being mindful of these common mistakes and taking steps to avoid them, you can ensure that you are on the right track towards achieving your weight loss goals. Remember to eat regular, balanced meals, stay hydrated, make healthy food choices, and prioritize sleep to support your weight loss efforts. With these tips in mind, you can successfully lose weight fast while maintaining your health and well-being.

Chapter 4: Overcoming Challenges

Dealing with Hunger Pangs

Dealing with hunger pangs is one of the biggest challenges when it comes to following a one meal a day (OMAD) diet for weight loss. It's natural to feel hungry when you're only eating one meal a day, but there are strategies you can use to manage those hunger pangs and stay on track with your weight loss goals.

One of the most important things to remember when dealing with hunger pangs on a one meal a day diet is to make sure that your one meal is balanced and nutritious. Including a good balance of protein, healthy fats, and fiber in your meal can help you feel full and satisfied for longer, reducing the likelihood of experiencing hunger pangs later in the day.

Another helpful tip for managing hunger pangs on a one meal a day diet is to stay hydrated. Sometimes our bodies mistake thirst for hunger, so drinking plenty of water throughout the day can help curb those hunger pangs and keep you feeling full between meals.

If you find yourself feeling hungry between meals, try distracting yourself with a non-food related activity, such as going for a walk, reading a book, or doing a puzzle. Keeping your mind occupied can help take your focus off of food and reduce the intensity of your hunger pangs.

Finally, remember that it's okay to feel a little hungry on a one meal a day diet. It's normal for your body to adjust to a new eating schedule, and some hunger pangs are to be expected. Just make sure to listen to your body and eat when you're truly hungry, rather than eating out of boredom or habit. With these strategies in mind, you can successfully navigate hunger pangs on a one meal a day diet and achieve your weight loss goals in a healthy way.

Managing Social Situations

Managing social situations can be one of the biggest challenges when you are trying to lose weight fast with the one meal a day approach. It's common to feel pressure from friends and family to eat more, especially during social gatherings or events. However, it's important to remember that your health and weight loss goals are top priorities. With the right strategies, you can navigate social situations without compromising your progress.

One key strategy for managing social situations is to plan ahead. Before attending a social gathering, think about what food options will be available and how you can stick to your one meal a day plan. Consider eating a small, protein-rich snack before the event to help curb your appetite and prevent overeating. You can also bring a healthy dish to share with others, ensuring that you have a nutritious option to enjoy.

Another important aspect of managing social situations is communication. Be open and honest with your friends and family about your weight loss goals and the reasons behind your one meal a day approach. By explaining your journey and the importance of sticking to your plan, you can gain their support and understanding. Additionally, don't be afraid to politely decline offers of food or drink that don't align with your goals.

Finding alternative ways to socialize that don't revolve around food can also be helpful when trying to lose weight fast with the one meal a day approach. Suggesting activities such as going for a walk, attending a fitness class, or meeting for a coffee instead of a meal can help shift the focus away from eating. This can also provide a new and enjoyable way to connect with others while staying on track with your weight loss goals.

Lastly, remember to be kind to yourself and practice self-compassion. It's okay to indulge occasionally or make exceptions in social situations, as long as you are mindful and make healthy choices the majority of the time. By finding a balance that works for you and staying committed to your goals, you can successfully navigate social situations while losing weight fast with the one meal a day approach.

Staying Motivated

Staying motivated is crucial when embarking on a weight loss journey, especially when following a plan like the One Meal a Day to Lose Weight method. It can be challenging to stick to a strict eating schedule and resist temptations, but with the right mindset and strategies, you can stay on track and achieve your goals.

One way to stay motivated is to set realistic and achievable goals for yourself. Instead of focusing on the end result, break down your weight loss journey into smaller milestones that you can celebrate along the way. This will help you stay motivated and inspired to continue making progress.

Another important aspect of staying motivated is to find a support system. Whether it's friends, family, or an online community, having people to cheer you on and hold you accountable can make a world of difference. Surround yourself with positive influences who understand your goals and are there to support you through the ups and downs of your weight loss journey.

It's also essential to focus on the non-scale victories along the way. Celebrate the improvements in your energy levels, mood, and overall health that come with making healthier choices and sticking to your one meal a day plan. Remember that weight loss is not just about the number on the scale, but about feeling better and living a healthier life.

Lastly, don't be too hard on yourself if you slip up or have a bad day. Remember that progress is not always linear, and setbacks are a natural part of any weight loss journey. Instead of giving up, use these setbacks as learning opportunities and motivation to keep pushing forward towards your goals. Stay positive, stay focused, and stay motivated on your journey to fast weight loss the healthy way.

Chapter 5: Maintaining Weight Loss and Long-Term Health

Transitioning to a Sustainable Eating Pattern

Transitioning to a sustainable eating pattern is crucial for long-term success in weight loss and overall health. While quick fixes may provide temporary results, they are often unsustainable and can lead to negative consequences in the long run. By focusing on creating a healthy and balanced eating pattern, you can not only achieve your weight loss goals but also maintain them over time.

One effective way to transition to a sustainable eating pattern is by adopting the practice of one meal a day (OMAD). OMAD allows you to consume all your daily calories in one sitting, which can help regulate your hunger hormones and promote fat burning. However, it is important to ensure that your one meal is nutritionally balanced and provides all the essential nutrients your body needs to function properly.

When transitioning to a sustainable eating pattern, it is important to focus on incorporating whole, nutrient-dense foods into your diet. These foods are rich in vitamins, minerals, and antioxidants, which can help support your overall health and weight loss goals. By choosing foods such as fruits, vegetables, whole grains, lean proteins, and healthy fats, you can fuel your body with the nutrients it needs to thrive.

In addition to focusing on the types of foods you eat, it is also important to pay attention to portion sizes and meal timing. Eating a balanced meal that includes all the essential nutrients in the right portions can help prevent overeating and promote satiety. Additionally, paying attention to when you eat can help regulate your metabolism and promote efficient digestion, which can aid in weight loss and overall health.

By making small, sustainable changes to your eating pattern, you can achieve your weight loss goals in a healthy and effective way. Remember that the key to long-term success is consistency and balance. By focusing on nourishing your body with whole, nutrient-dense foods and practicing mindful eating habits, you can create a sustainable eating pattern that supports your weight loss journey and overall health.

Incorporating Exercise for Optimal Results

Incorporating exercise into your weight loss journey is crucial for achieving optimal results. While switching to a one meal a day (OMAD) approach can help you shed pounds quickly, adding physical activity to your routine can further enhance your progress. In this subchapter, we will explore the benefits of exercise for weight loss and provide tips on how to incorporate it into your OMAD lifestyle.

Regular exercise not only burns calories but also boosts your metabolism, making it easier to achieve your weight loss goals. By engaging in physical activity, you can increase your energy expenditure and create a calorie deficit, which is key to losing weight. Additionally, exercise helps to build muscle, which can further enhance your metabolism and improve your overall body composition.

When incorporating exercise into your OMAD routine, it's important to choose activities that you enjoy and that fit your lifestyle. Whether it's going for a brisk walk, hitting the gym, or practicing yoga, finding a form of exercise that you look forward to can make it easier to stick to your routine. Remember, consistency is key when it comes to achieving long-term weight loss success.

To maximize the benefits of exercise, consider incorporating both cardiovascular and strength training workouts into your routine. Cardiovascular exercises, such as running or cycling, can help you burn calories and improve your cardiovascular health. Strength training exercises, on the other hand, can help you build muscle and increase your metabolism, leading to greater fat loss over time.

In conclusion, incorporating exercise into your OMAD weight loss journey can help you achieve optimal results in a healthy way. By finding activities that you enjoy, staying consistent, and incorporating both cardiovascular and strength training exercises, you can boost your metabolism, burn more calories, and improve your overall fitness. Remember, weight loss is a journey, and by adding exercise to your routine, you can enhance your results and achieve your goals faster.

Monitoring Your Progress and Adjusting as Needed

As you embark on your journey to fast weight loss through the one meal a day approach, it is crucial to monitor your progress regularly. Keeping track of your weight, measurements, and how you feel can provide valuable insight into how your body is responding to this new eating pattern. By tracking your progress, you can identify patterns, successes, and areas for improvement. This information will allow you to make informed decisions about your diet and lifestyle moving forward.

One effective way to monitor your progress is by keeping a food journal. Write down everything you eat and drink throughout the day, as well as how you feel after each meal. This will help you identify any trigger foods or patterns that may be hindering your weight loss progress. Additionally, tracking your food intake can help you stay accountable and make conscious choices about what you are putting into your body.

In addition to keeping a food journal, regularly weighing yourself and taking measurements can provide concrete data on your progress. Remember that weight loss is not always linear and can fluctuate due to various factors such as water retention, muscle gain, and hormonal changes. By tracking your weight and measurements over time, you can see the overall trend and make adjustments as needed to stay on track towards your weight loss goals.

It is important to listen to your body and make adjustments as needed. If you are feeling fatigued, sluggish, or not seeing the results you desire, it may be time to reevaluate your one meal a day plan. Consider consulting with a healthcare professional or nutritionist to ensure you are getting all the essential nutrients your body needs. They can provide guidance on how to adjust your meal plan to better support your weight loss goals while maintaining optimal health.

In conclusion, monitoring your progress and adjusting as needed is a crucial component of fast weight loss through the one meal a day approach. By keeping track of your progress, making informed decisions about your diet and lifestyle, and listening to your body, you can achieve sustainable and healthy weight loss results. Remember, everyone's journey is unique, so be patient with yourself and stay committed to your goals. With dedication and perseverance, you can reach your desired weight and improve your overall health and well-being.

Chapter 6: Success Stories and Testimonials

Real-Life Experiences with OMAD

Many people have tried the OMAD (One Meal a Day) approach to weight loss and have seen incredible results. One individual, Sarah, shared her experience with OMAD and how it helped her shed pounds quickly and in a healthy way. She mentioned that by only eating one meal a day, she was able to control her calorie intake and avoid mindless snacking throughout the day. Sarah found that she had more energy and mental clarity while following the OMAD approach, which made it easier for her to stick to her weight loss goals.

Another person, John, also had success with OMAD and was able to lose over 20 pounds in just a few months. He mentioned that by eating one large, nutrient-dense meal each day, he felt full and satisfied, which helped him avoid overeating or giving into cravings. John found that OMAD not only helped him lose weight, but also improved his digestion and overall health. He emphasized the importance of choosing whole, nutritious foods for his one meal to ensure he was getting all the essential nutrients his body needed.

For many individuals, the convenience of OMAD is a major selling point. Rachel, a busy working mom, found that following the OMAD approach allowed her to save time and money on meal prep and planning. She mentioned that she no longer had to worry about packing multiple meals and snacks for the day, as she could simply focus on preparing one nutritious meal each evening. Rachel also found that OMAD helped her break free from emotional eating habits, as she was more mindful and intentional about her food choices during her one meal each day.

One common concern about OMAD is whether it is sustainable in the long term. However, many individuals have found that they can continue to follow the OMAD approach even after reaching their weight loss goals. Mark, who lost over 50 pounds with OMAD, mentioned that he has been able to maintain his weight by incorporating occasional fasting days or adjusting his meal size based on his activity level. He emphasized the importance of listening to his body and making adjustments as needed to ensure he stays healthy and happy.

In conclusion, real-life experiences with OMAD show that this approach to weight loss can be effective, sustainable, and healthy when done correctly. By focusing on nutrient-dense foods, listening to your body's hunger cues, and being mindful about your eating habits, you can achieve fast weight loss results with OMAD. Whether you are a busy professional, a stay-at-home parent, or someone looking to break free from unhealthy eating patterns, giving OMAD a try may be the solution you've been looking for to reach your weight loss goals in a healthy way.

Tips and Tricks from Those Who Have Achieved Success

In this subchapter, we will explore some valuable tips and tricks from individuals who have successfully achieved their weight loss goals using the One Meal a Day (OMAD) approach. These insights can serve as inspiration and guidance for those who are looking to embark on their own weight loss journey.

One important tip that many successful individuals swear by is to plan ahead. By preparing your one meal in advance, you can ensure that you are making healthy choices and avoid the temptation of reaching for unhealthy snacks or fast food. Planning your meals also helps you stay on track with your calorie intake and ensures that you are getting all the necessary nutrients your body needs.

Another key trick to success with OMAD is to listen to your body. Pay attention to hunger cues and eat only when you are truly hungry. Avoid emotional eating or eating out of boredom, as this can lead to overeating and sabotage your weight loss efforts. By listening to your body's signals, you can develop a better understanding of your hunger and fullness cues, which is essential for long-term success with OMAD.

Furthermore, many successful individuals emphasize the importance of staying hydrated. Drinking plenty of water throughout the day can help curb cravings, boost metabolism, and promote overall health. Aim to drink at least eight glasses of water a day, and consider incorporating herbal teas or infused water for added variety and flavor. Staying hydrated can also help prevent overeating during your one meal, as thirst is often mistaken for hunger.

Additionally, it is crucial to incorporate regular physical activity into your routine. Many successful individuals combine OMAD with a consistent exercise regimen to maximize weight loss results and improve overall health. Whether it's going for a brisk walk, hitting the gym, or engaging in a home workout, finding an activity that you enjoy and can stick to is key. Exercise not only burns calories but also helps build muscle, boost metabolism, and improve mood, all of which are essential for successful weight loss with OMAD.

Lastly, one of the most important tips from those who have achieved success with OMAD is to be patient and consistent. Weight loss takes time, and it's essential to stay committed to your goals even when progress seems slow. Celebrate small victories along the way, and remember that every healthy choice you make brings you one step closer to your desired outcome. By implementing these tips and tricks from individuals who have successfully lost weight with OMAD, you can set yourself up for success and achieve your weight loss goals in a healthy and sustainable way.

Inspiring Stories of Transformation

In this subchapter, we will delve into some inspiring stories of transformation from individuals who have successfully adopted the One Meal a Day (OMAD) approach to lose weight in a healthy way. These stories serve as a source of motivation and encouragement for those looking to embark on their own weight loss journey using the OMAD method.

One such inspiring story is that of Sarah, a busy working mother who struggled with her weight for years. After discovering the OMAD approach, Sarah decided to give it a try and was amazed by the results. By sticking to one nutritious meal a day and making healthier food choices, Sarah was able to shed the excess pounds and regain her confidence. Her story is a testament to the power of determination and consistency when it comes to achieving weight loss goals.

Another inspiring transformation story comes from John, a middle-aged man who had been battling obesity for most of his adult life. Tired of crash diets and fad weight loss programs that never seemed to work, John decided to try the OMAD approach as a last resort. To his surprise, he found that eating one balanced meal a day not only helped him lose weight quickly but also improved his overall health and energy levels. John's story serves as a reminder that sustainable weight loss is possible with the right mindset and approach.

For Mary, a college student struggling to balance her studies and social life while also trying to lose weight, the OMAD approach was a game-changer. By focusing on one healthy meal a day and avoiding mindless snacking, Mary was able to achieve her weight loss goals without feeling deprived or restricted. Her story illustrates that it is possible to achieve fast weight loss in a healthy way by making simple yet effective changes to your daily eating habits.

These inspiring stories of transformation highlight the effectiveness of the OMAD approach for fast and healthy weight loss. By adopting this method and making smart food choices, individuals like Sarah, John, and Mary were able to achieve their weight loss goals and improve their overall well-being. Their journeys serve as a reminder that with dedication, consistency, and the right approach, anyone can achieve their desired weight loss results using the One Meal a Day strategy.

Chapter 7: Frequently Asked Questions

Can I Drink Coffee or Tea During the Fasting Period?

One common question that often arises when discussing fasting for weight loss is whether or not it is permissible to consume coffee or tea during the fasting period. The good news is that both coffee and tea are generally considered acceptable to drink while fasting. In fact, many people find that these beverages can actually help curb hunger and make it easier to stick to their fasting regimen.

When it comes to coffee, black coffee is the best option to drink while fasting. This means no sugar, cream, or any other additives. Some people also choose to drink their coffee with a splash of unsweetened almond or coconut milk, which is generally okay as long as it is kept to a minimum. The caffeine in coffee can help boost metabolism and increase fat burning, making it a popular choice for those looking to lose weight.

Tea is another great option for those fasting for weight loss. Like coffee, it is best to drink tea without any added sugar or milk. Green tea, in particular, has been shown to have numerous health benefits, including aiding in weight loss. It is packed with antioxidants and can help boost metabolism, making it a great choice for those looking to shed pounds.

It is important to note that while coffee and tea are generally acceptable to drink during the fasting period, it is best to limit consumption to avoid disrupting the fasting process. Both beverages can have a diuretic effect, so it is important to stay hydrated by drinking plenty of water throughout the day. Additionally, some people may find that drinking too much caffeine on an empty stomach can lead to jitters or an upset stomach, so it is best to listen to your body and adjust your intake accordingly.

In conclusion, coffee and tea can be great additions to a fasting regimen for weight loss. They can help curb hunger, boost metabolism, and provide numerous health benefits. Just be sure to drink them without added sugar or milk, and listen to your body to determine the right amount for you. With the right approach, incorporating coffee and tea into your fasting routine can help you achieve your weight loss goals in a healthy and sustainable way.

Is OMAD Safe for Everyone?

The concept of eating just one meal a day, also known as OMAD, has gained popularity in recent years as a way to promote fast weight loss. But is this extreme form of intermittent fasting safe for everyone? While OMAD can be an effective way to shed pounds quickly, it may not be suitable for everyone, especially those with certain health conditions or dietary needs.

One of the main concerns with OMAD is the potential for nutrient deficiencies. Eating just one meal a day can make it difficult to consume all the necessary vitamins, minerals, and macronutrients your body needs to function properly. This can lead to fatigue, weakness, and other health issues if not managed properly. It is important to consult with a healthcare professional before starting an OMAD regimen to ensure you are getting all the nutrients your body needs.

Another potential risk of OMAD is the impact on metabolism. Some people may experience a decrease in metabolism when eating only one meal a day, which can make it harder to lose weight in the long run. Additionally, drastic changes in eating patterns can disrupt your body's natural hunger and fullness cues, leading to overeating or undereating in the long term.

For individuals with certain medical conditions, such as diabetes or eating disorders, OMAD may not be safe or recommended. People with diabetes need to carefully monitor their blood sugar levels and may require more frequent meals to manage their condition. Those with a history of eating disorders may find that restricting their eating to just one meal a day can trigger unhealthy behaviors and thoughts around food.

In conclusion, while OMAD can be a helpful tool for fast weight loss, it may not be suitable for everyone. It is important to consider your individual health needs and consult with a healthcare professional before starting an OMAD regimen. If you do decide to try OMAD, be sure to listen to your body, eat a well-balanced meal, and monitor your overall health and well-being. Remember, weight loss should always be approached in a safe and sustainable way.

How Quickly Can I Expect to See Results?

When embarking on a weight loss journey, one of the most common questions people have is, "How quickly can I expect to see results?" The answer to this question can vary depending on a number of factors, including your starting weight, body composition, and adherence to the One Meal a Day (OMAD) approach. However, many people find that they start to see results within the first week of following a OMAD plan.

One of the key benefits of the OMAD approach is that it can lead to rapid weight loss. By consuming all of your daily calories in one meal, you are able to create a calorie deficit that can help you shed pounds quickly. Many people find that they start to see the numbers on the scale drop within the first few days of following a OMAD plan. This initial weight loss is often due to a reduction in water weight, but it can be a motivating factor to keep going.

In addition to weight loss, many people also report other positive changes in their bodies when following a OMAD plan. Some people find that their energy levels increase, their digestion improves, and they experience mental clarity and focus. These changes can occur relatively quickly, sometimes within the first few days of following a OMAD plan. This can be an added incentive to stick with the plan and continue on your weight loss journey.

It's important to remember that everyone's body is different, and results may vary from person to person. Some people may see rapid weight loss right away, while others may take longer to see significant changes. It's important to be patient and stay consistent with your OMAD plan in order to see the best results. Remember, slow and steady progress is often more sustainable in the long run than rapid weight loss that is difficult to maintain.

Overall, while results may vary, many people find that they start to see positive changes in their bodies relatively quickly when following a One Meal a Day approach. By creating a calorie deficit and sticking to a healthy meal plan, you can expect to see results within the first week or two of following a OMAD plan. Keep in mind that consistency is key, and staying committed to your goals can help you achieve the results you desire in a healthy way.

Chapter 8: Conclusion

Recap of Key Points

In this subchapter, we will recap the key points discussed in "The One Meal Solution: Fast Weight Loss the Healthy Way" for those who want to lose weight fast through the practice of One Meal a Day (OMAD) in a healthy manner.

The first key point to remember is the importance of choosing nutrient-dense foods for your one meal. It is crucial to make sure that you are getting all the necessary vitamins, minerals, and macronutrients in that single meal to fuel your body properly. This means including plenty of fruits, vegetables, lean proteins, and whole grains in your meal.

Another important point to keep in mind is portion control. Just because you are only eating one meal a day does not give you free reign to overeat. It is still important to listen to your body's hunger cues and stop eating when you are satisfied. Overeating, even in one meal, can sabotage your weight loss efforts.

Hydration is key when practicing OMAD. Make sure to drink plenty of water throughout the day to stay hydrated and keep your body functioning optimally. Herbal teas and black coffee are also great options to help curb hunger and keep you feeling full between meals.

Consistency is key when it comes to seeing results with OMAD. Stick to your one meal a day schedule and try to eat at the same time each day to help regulate your body's hunger signals. Remember, weight loss takes time and patience, so don't get discouraged if you don't see results right away.

Lastly, it is important to listen to your body and make adjustments as needed. If you are feeling excessively hungry or fatigued, it may be a sign that OMAD is not the best approach for you. It is important to prioritize your health and well-being above all else when it comes to weight loss.

Final Thoughts and Encouragement for Your Weight Loss Journey

As you embark on your weight loss journey with the goal of losing weight fast, it is important to remember that the key to success lies in consistency and perseverance. Adopting the one meal a day approach can be a powerful tool in helping you achieve your weight loss goals, but it is essential to approach it in a healthy way. By focusing on nutrient-dense foods and listening to your body's hunger cues, you can fuel your body effectively while still creating a calorie deficit to promote weight loss.

One of the most important things to keep in mind as you navigate your weight loss journey is to be patient with yourself. Sustainable weight loss takes time and effort, and there will inevitably be ups and downs along the way. It is important to celebrate your successes, no matter how small, and to learn from any setbacks you may encounter. Remember that every step you take towards your goal, no matter how small, is a step in the right direction.

In addition to being patient with yourself, it is also important to be kind to yourself throughout your weight loss journey. Losing weight can be a challenging and emotional process, and it is important to practice self-care and self-compassion along the way. Treat yourself with the same kindness and understanding that you would offer to a friend going through a similar journey, and remember that you are worthy of love and respect no matter where you are in your weight loss journey.

As you continue on your weight loss journey, it can be helpful to seek support from others who are going through similar experiences. Whether it is joining a support group, working with a weight loss coach, or simply confiding in a trusted friend or family member, having a support system in place can make a world of difference. Surround yourself with people who uplift and encourage you, and who understand the challenges and triumphs that come with losing weight.

In conclusion, your weight loss journey is a personal and transformative experience that has the potential to change your life for the better. By approaching it with patience, kindness, and support, you can achieve your weight loss goals in a healthy and sustainable way. Remember that you are capable of achieving anything you set your mind to, and that you deserve to live a happy, healthy, and fulfilling life. Keep pushing forward, stay true to your goals, and trust in yourself and your ability to succeed. You've got this!

Recipe 1: Grilled Chicken and Veggie Bowl

Ingredients:

- 1 large chicken breast
- 1 bell pepper, sliced
- 1 zucchini, sliced
- 1 cup cherry tomatoes
- 1/2 cup quinoa or brown rice
- 2 tbsp olive oil
- Salt and pepper to taste
- 1 tsp garlic powder
- 1 tsp paprika
- 1 avocado, sliced

Instructions:

1. **Cook the Quinoa/Rice**: Prepare quinoa or brown rice according to package instructions.
2. **Marinate the Chicken**: In a bowl, mix olive oil, salt, pepper, garlic powder, and paprika. Coat the chicken breast with the mixture.
3. **Grill the Chicken**: Heat a grill or grill pan over medium-high heat. Grill the chicken for about 6-7 minutes per side, or until fully cooked.
4. **Cook the Veggies**: In a separate pan, sauté bell pepper, zucchini, and cherry tomatoes in olive oil until tender.
5. **Assemble the Bowl**: Slice the grilled chicken and place it over a bed of quinoa or brown rice. Add the cooked veggies and sliced avocado on top.
6. **Serve**: Enjoy your hearty and nutritious bowl!

Recipe 2: Salmon and Sweet Potato

Ingredients:

- 1 salmon fillet
- 1 large sweet potato
- 1 cup broccoli florets
- 1 tbsp olive oil
- 1 lemon
- Salt and pepper to taste
- 1 tsp dried dill

Instructions:

1. **Prepare the Sweet Potato**: Preheat the oven to 400°F (200°C). Slice the sweet potato into rounds, drizzle with olive oil, and season with salt and pepper. Roast in the oven for about 25-30 minutes, or until tender.
2. **Cook the Salmon**: Season the salmon fillet with salt, pepper, and dried dill. Place it on a baking sheet and squeeze half a lemon over it. Bake in the oven for about 15-20 minutes, or until the salmon flakes easily with a fork.
3. **Steam the Broccoli**: While the salmon and sweet potatoes are cooking, steam the broccoli florets until tender.
4. **Assemble the Plate**: Place the roasted sweet potatoes and steamed broccoli on a plate. Add the cooked salmon fillet on top.
5. **Serve**: Garnish with a slice of lemon and enjoy your delicious and balanced meal!

Recipe 3: Beef and Veggie Stir-Fry

Ingredients:

- 200g lean beef strips
- 1 bell pepper, sliced
- 1 carrot, julienned
- 1 cup snap peas
- 1 small onion, sliced
- 2 cloves garlic, minced
- 2 tbsp soy sauce
- 1 tbsp oyster sauce
- 1 tbsp olive oil
- 1 tsp sesame oil
- 1/2 cup jasmine rice

Instructions:

1. **Cook the Rice**: Prepare jasmine rice according to package instructions.
2. **Marinate the Beef**: In a bowl, mix soy sauce, oyster sauce, and minced garlic. Add the beef strips and let them marinate for at least 15 minutes.

3. **Cook the Beef**: Heat olive oil in a large pan over medium-high heat. Add the beef strips and cook until browned. Remove from the pan and set aside.
4. **Cook the Veggies**: In the same pan, add a bit more olive oil if needed. Sauté the onion, bell pepper, carrot, and snap peas until tender.
5. **Combine and Serve**: Add the beef back into the pan with the veggies. Stir in sesame oil and cook for an additional 2-3 minutes. Serve the stir-fry over a bed of jasmine rice.

Recipe 4: Vegetarian Buddha Bowl

Ingredients:

- 1/2 cup chickpeas, cooked
- 1 sweet potato, cubed
- 1 cup spinach leaves
- 1/2 avocado, sliced
- 1/4 cup hummus
- 1 tbsp olive oil
- Salt and pepper to taste
- 1 tsp cumin
- 1/2 tsp paprika
- 1/2 cup quinoa

Instructions:

1. **Cook the Quinoa**: Prepare quinoa according to package instructions.
2. **Roast the Sweet Potato**: Preheat the oven to 400°F (200°C). Toss the sweet potato cubes with olive oil, salt, pepper, cumin, and paprika. Roast in the oven for about 25-30 minutes, or until tender.
3. **Prepare the Chickpeas**: If using canned chickpeas, drain and rinse them. If using dried chickpeas, cook them according to package instructions.
4. **Assemble the Bowl**: In a bowl, arrange the cooked quinoa, roasted sweet potatoes, chickpeas, spinach leaves, and sliced avocado.
5. **Add Hummus**: Add a dollop of hummus on top for added flavor and creaminess.
6. **Serve**: Enjoy your nutrient-packed vegetarian Buddha bowl!

Recipe 5: Shrimp and Avocado Salad

Ingredients:

- 200g shrimp, peeled and deveined
- 1 avocado, diced
- 1 cucumber, diced
- 1 cup cherry tomatoes, halved
- 1/4 red onion, thinly sliced
- 2 tbsp olive oil
- 1 tbsp lemon juice
- Salt and pepper to taste
- 1/2 tsp paprika
- Fresh parsley or cilantro for garnish

Instructions:

1. **Cook the Shrimp**: Heat 1 tbsp of olive oil in a pan over medium heat. Add the shrimp, season with salt, pepper, and paprika, and cook until pink and fully cooked (about 2-3 minutes per side). Remove from heat and let cool slightly.
2. **Prepare the Vegetables**: In a large bowl, combine the diced avocado, cucumber, cherry tomatoes, and red onion.
3. **Dress the Salad**: Drizzle the vegetables with the remaining olive oil and lemon juice. Toss gently to combine.
4. **Assemble the Salad**: Add the cooked shrimp to the vegetable mixture and toss gently.
5. **Garnish and Serve**: Garnish with fresh parsley or cilantro and enjoy your refreshing shrimp and avocado salad.

Recipe 6: Spaghetti Squash with Turkey Bolognese

Ingredients:

- 1 spaghetti squash
- 200g ground turkey
- 1 can (14 oz) crushed tomatoes
- 1 small onion, diced
- 2 cloves garlic, minced
- 1 carrot, grated
- 2 tbsp olive oil
- 1 tsp dried oregano
- 1 tsp dried basil
- Salt and pepper to taste
- Grated Parmesan cheese for serving (optional)

Instructions:

1. **Prepare the Spaghetti Squash**: Preheat the oven to 400°F (200°C). Cut the spaghetti squash in half lengthwise and remove the seeds. Drizzle with olive oil, season with salt and pepper, and place cut-side down on a baking sheet. Roast for about 40 minutes, or until tender.
2. **Cook the Turkey Bolognese**: While the squash is roasting, heat 2 tbsp of olive oil in a large pan over medium heat. Add the onion and garlic and sauté until fragrant. Add the ground turkey and cook until browned.
3. **Add Vegetables and Tomatoes**: Add the grated carrot, crushed tomatoes, oregano, basil, salt, and pepper to the pan. Simmer for about 20 minutes, stirring occasionally, until the sauce has thickened.
4. **Prepare the Spaghetti Squash Noodles**: Once the squash is done roasting, use a fork to scrape out the flesh into spaghetti-like strands.
5. **Assemble the Dish**: Divide the spaghetti squash noodles between plates and top with the turkey Bolognese sauce.

6. **Serve**: Sprinkle with grated Parmesan cheese, if desired, and enjoy your healthy and delicious meal.

Recipe 7: Tofu and Vegetable Stir-Fry

Ingredients:

- 200g firm tofu, cubed
- 1 red bell pepper, sliced
- 1 cup broccoli florets
- 1 carrot, julienned
- 1/2 cup snap peas
- 2 tbsp soy sauce
- 1 tbsp sesame oil
- 1 tbsp olive oil
- 2 cloves garlic, minced
- 1 tsp ginger, minced
- 1 tsp cornstarch
- 1/4 cup vegetable broth
- Cooked brown rice for serving

Instructions:

1. **Prepare the Tofu**: Press the tofu to remove excess moisture, then cut into cubes. In a bowl, mix 1 tbsp soy sauce and cornstarch, then toss the tofu cubes in the mixture.
2. **Cook the Tofu**: Heat olive oil in a pan over medium-high heat. Add the tofu and cook until golden brown on all sides. Remove from the pan and set aside.
3. **Cook the Vegetables**: In the same pan, add sesame oil, garlic, and ginger. Sauté until fragrant. Add the bell pepper, broccoli, carrot, and snap peas, and stir-fry until tender.
4. **Combine and Serve**: Add the tofu back to the pan along with the remaining soy sauce and vegetable broth. Stir to combine and cook for an additional 2-3 minutes.
5. **Serve**: Serve the tofu and vegetable stir-fry over a bed of brown rice.

Recipe 8: Lentil and Vegetable Stew

Ingredients:

- 1 cup green or brown lentils, rinsed
- 1 onion, diced
- 2 cloves garlic, minced
- 2 carrots, sliced
- 2 celery stalks, sliced
- 1 zucchini, diced
- 1 can (14 oz) diced tomatoes
- 4 cups vegetable broth
- 1 tbsp olive oil
- 1 tsp cumin
- 1 tsp paprika
- Salt and pepper to taste
- Fresh parsley for garnish

Instructions:

1. **Sauté the Aromatics**: In a large pot, heat olive oil over medium heat. Add the onion and garlic and sauté until softened.
2. **Add Vegetables**: Add the carrots, celery, and zucchini. Cook for another 5 minutes.
3. **Add Lentils and Broth**: Stir in the lentils, diced tomatoes, vegetable broth, cumin, paprika, salt, and pepper. Bring to a boil.
4. **Simmer**: Reduce the heat and let the stew simmer for about 30-40 minutes, or until the lentils and vegetables are tender.
5. **Serve**: Garnish with fresh parsley and enjoy your hearty and nutritious lentil stew.